The *Seven Key*

Fundamentals to

TRANSFORMING YOUR

BODY

**DON'T WASTE ANYMORE MORE
TIME AND MONEY. USE A WORKING
SYSTEM AND STRATEGY.**

PAUL STEIGER

Founder of Steiger Fitness

Facebook * Instagram *Website

Cover design and layout by Ron Scott
Cover Model Paul Steiger
Cover Photo by Wainwright Images
Editing Acknowledgments: Kristina Canady and
Kathleen Payne

Book content design/formatting by Kristina Canady

Legal Disclaimer

The information contained in this book is the opinion of the author and is based on the author's personal experiences and observations. The author does not assume any liability whatsoever for the use of or inability to use any or all information contained in this book, and accepts no responsibility for any loss or damages of any kind that may be incurred by the reader as a result of actions arising from the use of information found in this book. Use this information at your own risk.

The author reserves the right to make any changes he deems necessary to future versions of the publication to ensure its accuracy.

WHAT CAN YOU EXPECT FROM THE SEVEN KEY FUNDAMENTALS TO TRANSFORMING YOUR BODY?

It is my goal to help you quickly learn my seven-step strategy to aid your current fat loss and muscle building routines. Throughout this book, I've incorporated new and unique ideas that can be applied to what you are currently doing and help increase your fitness outcomes tremendously.

Before we begin, let's make sure that we are on the same page. To achieve anything great or worth doing, it will take hard work, and the changes may not come easy. No one can promise an overnight success plan. It is my hope that by outlining these strategic tools that you can apply to your current program, you will gain maximum benefits, and perform at peak level. If you think you have what it takes and want to boost success rates, then let's get started.

CONTENTS

- Don't waste your money

- The six supplements you really need

- Supplements supplement your diet, not replace

- Your muscles need resistance and constant work

- Work hard

- Attention to each body part

- What is cardio?

- Different types of cardio

- Benefits of cardio

- Your muscles need rest to grow

- Stretching your muscles

INTRODUCTION

After speaking with numerous people about their gym routines, their diet, or lack thereof, and how many hours they waste at the gym, I was inspired to write this book. My passion only grew as I watched others struggle with the lack of the necessary knowledge to be successful. I honestly felt frustrated for them and still do.

Those who show up to workout get an 'A' for effort because that is half the battle. I also salute those who put in one, two, or for the overachiever, maybe even three hours at the gym. That alone takes dedication. Yes, you see some results but not to the full degree that you truly want or deserve after all of that determination. Week after week, you work your ass off, yet the results you labor so hard for aren't coming through. Why is that? Wouldn't you love it if every hour you spent at the gym helped you reach your set goals and showed you vast improvements week after week?

Keep reading, I will explain how to see those payouts...

First, let me tell you a little bit about myself. After all, you decided to read my book, or at least read this far, which I appreciate, but why keep going? Great question. I would be wondering the same exact thing, and would want to know a little bit about the author before spending the time to read his or her material.

So here it goes. My name is Paul. I am an entrepreneur, fitness model, and personal trainer. Beyond all the fancy titles, I'm just another guy who decided to stop living a mediocre life and change by improving my physique, my health, and my mindset.

At the age of sixteen, I started working

out and have been going to the gym ever since. In the past fifteen years, I've only taken off about a month at the most. Being curious and open to all of the different fitness techniques, I have done just about every workout and tried almost every supplement. Even with all of that, my results weren't improving. My physique was not changing, and I was just another gym rat wasting time.

Even though I knew diet played a huge role, I unfortunately didn't have the right mindset or motivation to actually follow through on the level needed. That's when I realized the biggest secret to success was one, hiring an expert or a coach, and two, focusing on controlling my mind.

After seeking out the right resources, and learning how to get my head in the game, I have accomplished more in the past year then I have over the past fifteen.

If I can do it, you can too, my friend, and I want to help.

The desired results will take hard work, dedication, and, with a little professional help, you will be able to achieve your fitness goals faster and more efficiently. What I have personally accomplished is completely attainable for you as well. Let me help you transform your physique and lifestyle by improving your diet, training, and mindset.

Many people are often quick to believe the worst, that they are the reason they can't achieve lasting results. The problem isn't with them, it's with their strategy. They think that the way to get into better shape is to exercise a couple times a week, and the results will come. Or, they've set out on an extreme mission to change their body, by going through numerous diets, workout routines, either found online or given by a friend, only to achieve a fraction of the results they anticipated. Another mental trap that can affect their tactic is falling for the opinions and advice by everyone in their circle who may play it off as being extremely simple. Their input centers around how one just needs to get off the couch, get motivated, snatch up a gym membership, get a trainer, eat healthy, and your goals of becoming fit and having the body you always wanted is just a couple months away.

This is a partial truth. More like five percent of the full picture. In this book, I will take you deeper into what crucial tips and tricks you need to know in order to maximize your hard work. We will also cover the most important thing you can do to help achieve your goals, which is pure tactic.

Throughout my journey, I have found seven critical areas that allowed me to find success on my quest to get the body I always dreamed of, I call it The Seven Fundamentals to Transforming Your Body. Let's jump right into chapter one, and let me begin with the first and most important fundamental, fueling your body.

CHAPTER 1 - FUELING YOUR BODY

Food, or as I like to call it, fuel, is your number one ally. Think of your body as a machine, and food as the fuel to run this machine. Let's say you have an 800hp Ferrari and a 200hp Kia. Which one should be faster? The Ferrari right? Sure, the math makes sense. But let's say the Ferrari has no fuel, and the Kia does. Now, which one is faster? I think you get the point.

Your body works the same way. It needs fuel to run. Even if you work hard in the gym for 3 hours lifting all of the weight, you are wasting your time if you're not properly fueling your body before and after. Frequently, guys come up to me at the gym and ask me how I do it.

I tell them I eat, I fuel my body.

They often say, "I eat, too, and I eat a lot. As a matter of fact, I'm going to Chipotle right after the gym."

My first thought is, "Not the same bro!" The food you get at any restaurant, which only takes 5-10 minutes to get in and out of, will not give you the necessary nutrients, or fuel your body requires to heal and grow from your workout.

Most people eat for pleasure. We are taught by society that eating is a social thing. It is unusual for the majority of people to eat based on what is useful for their bodies. Let's be honest, you usually eat what tastes good, right? This is a terrible way of treating your body. All you are doing is satisfying your tastes buds, and at the same time, ignoring every other part of your body's needs during this process.

There are three essential macronutrients needed in each meal. Proteins, carbohydrates, and fats. Now, I'm not going to lecture about what protein is, the difference between good and bad fats, or what carbohydrates are and how much to eat of them. But this stuff is super important so...

actually, I lied to you.

I am definitely going to tell you about these three vital fuel sources. We will cover which ones you want, which ones you need to stay away from, and the right amount of each. Many of you might already have a general idea on these and how to use them toward transforming your body. However, we will review them together to make sure all of the basics are covered.

Protein

Let's start with protein because it is the easiest to get a grasp on. Protein is crucial for your body because it helps your metabolism run at a faster rate, stabilizes blood sugar, and is an important key factor in building and repairing tissue and muscles. You consume protein every day, but the real question is, are you getting protein from sources that are good for your body and will genuinely help with your transformation goals? For example, a McDonald's Big Mac has 26grams of protein. That is a good amount of protein, but it also contains high amounts of fat and other additives that can have negative effects.

There are many sources of protein, but I'm going to stick to the basic options that will fuel your body and not destroy it over time. The protein sources that are nutritious and the most helpful in your body transformation quest are as follows:

-Chicken breast (skinless)

-99% fat free ground turkey

-97% fat free ground beef

-High quality steak (like a sirloin tip side that has little visible marbling, and mainly muscle)

-White fish (like Tilapia, Cod, or Halibut)

-Egg whites

-Protein powders mixed with water not milk and with low sugar and fat.

Before we continue, I hope you eat meat. If not, please consult vegan or vegetarian resource materials to find substitutes for animal protein. I'm not too familiar with plant based dieting.

That being said, let's get back to meat. I like to keep this as simple as possible. Personally, I primarily consume white meat from poultry, such as chicken breast and ground turkey. I'm not a fan of beef or fish. A combination of the above will work as long you stick to those sources of protein and eat the right amounts.

I eat at least 40 grams of protein per meal, and 6 meals total per day. That is about 240 grams of protein per day. This may seem like a lot, but remember, the goal is to build muscle, and your muscles need protein to grow. I weigh about 180lbs, so these are my numbers. A guy who weighs 200+ pounds will need to consume more. It is all a numbers game and you can do the math once you have the basics down of what to plug into your calculations. We could go deeper into what protein is, how it breaks down to its amino acid composition, and all the science behind it, but let's just keep it straightforward:

Protein builds and replenishes muscles. It is mandatory for muscle growth.

Carbohydrates

Now that we've briefly discussed protein, let's talk about the one macronutrient that most people have a love-hate relationship with: carbohydrates. Actually, who am I kidding, let's be honest – everyone loves carbs. Carbohydrates are your main source of energy, and they come from delicious foods like pasta, rice, breads, fruits, vegetables, and dairy products. Your body breaks down these foods into something called glucose. Glucose is basically sugar that can either give you immediate energy or your body can store it to be used for energy later.

Once again, I'm not going to get into extensive scientific explanation of carbs, I just want to cover the basics. Now that we know it gives us energy and our body needs it, how do we know which carbs are the right ones, which to stay away from, and the correct amounts to consume? Perfect question, I'm glad you asked.

The type of carbs that you eat will be more important than the amounts consumed, but if you want to gain lean muscle, we want to make sure you don't eat too many or not enough.

Before I get into crazy math with carbs, let's start with the easy part first: the good vs the bad. Bad carbs are foods such as white bread, pastries, sodas, milk, popcorn, cookies, pastas, cakes, and pies just to name a few. Yeah, I know, all the good stuff right? But remember, we are fueling our bodies, not feeding our taste buds even if that feels better. Are you done dreaming and salivating about cakes and pies? I hope so, because now we need to focus on the good carbs. It's important to learn to love them instead of the amazing and heavenly tasting garbage food we just finished talking about.

Good carbs are going to come from foods such as sweet potatoes (not fries but cooked or baked), white rice or brown rice (even though brown rice is a better option, eating white rice will not keep you off track), black beans or other legumes, vegetables (I know everyone's favorite), and fruit.

Let's pause for a moment – fruit has a high sugar content, we need to watch the quantity of that too. Yes, it is natural sugar, but eating more than necessary is going to take away from your progress. We will go over sugar and how to manage it in more depth later. Typically, I eat fruit in my oatmeal for breakfast so it gives me the morning energy I need, and then my body burns it away throughout the day.

Carbs are great for our bodies, and we love them. It's important that we understand them, thoroughly, and have awareness on properly managing carbs throughout our diets.

Fats

The third food source we are going to talk about is fats. What are fats? Are fats bad for you all around? Are there any fats that are good for you or useful to your body? Excellent questions, let's discuss them.

Fats provide you with energy, absorb nutrients, and maintain your body temperature.

Fats are an important part of your daily diet. With that being said, it is important that we consume fat in our diet to make sure our bodies can take advantage of these functions.

Now, just because fat is important to consume, you don't have the green light to go eat all of the mouthwatering fats you want. We know the fat you want to eat, it's the fat I want to eat too, trust me. That's when we have to remember we are fueling our bodies, not feeding our taste buds.

What are bad fats? There are two types of fats that are bad for you; they are called saturated fats and trans fats. Fats that are unhealthy or unnecessary to fuel your body can be found in animal products such as meat, milk, cheese, butter, and cream. You will also find plenty of bad fats in fast food and processed products.

As mentioned above, meat can also have fat in it that is not good for us, yet I told you when we talked about protein that we need to eat meat to grow our muscles. So, now what? Well, the good thing about meat is, there are some that don't have high amounts of bad fat.

For example, skinless chicken breast, and 99% fat free ground turkey will have extremely low amounts of fat. That is also why I choose to use them as my foundational protein. I'm not a fan of fish, which is why I usually avoid talking about it, but it is also a very good lean source of protein. If you like fish, that is awesome, eat up. Other meats like beef and pork are typically the highest in saturated fat so try to stay away from those as much as possible.

Another terrible source of fat is hydrogenated oils. These would be oils you find in most junk foods and fast foods. Also, it is common in peanut butter that is not natural, as well as margarine. Absolutely make sure that your food is not made with hydrogenated oils.

It is easier to avoid these fats and other harmful additives if you cook your own meals. This is a tip that I highly recommend to everyone I talk to as well. By prepping your own meals, you know exactly what goes in and from what sources.

Sugar

We started out discussing three primary food sources; however, there is one more little pesky substance I want to discuss with you. This one is detrimental to your diet. What am I talking about? I'm talking about sugar.

Technically sugar is a carbohydrate that also dissolves in your body. There are many different types of sugars. Good sugars are going to be the ones you get from natural sources such as fruits, some vegetables, beans, nuts, and whole grain. Now, I did mention not to eat too many fruits in a day because of the high sugar levels. Even though these sugars are not necessarily bad for you, they still have the capability to throw you off track when you are trying to achieve transformation of your body.

When you think of sugar, you are

probably thinking of table sugar, those tiny little crystals or the ground down, white chalky powder form. Most people don't sit there and eat spoonful's of sugar by itself; so let's discuss the hidden sugars that you don't even know you are consuming.

Or maybe you do eat spoonful's of sugar, I don't know. Hopefully, after you read this book, however, you will change that immediately.

Anyway, back to the sneaky, hidden, and terrible for you sugars... What are they? Sugars that you want to stay away from are the ones found in most of the foods you probably enjoy the most. They are added to foods during processing, cooking, or like I mentioned earlier, crystals or powdered sugars found in almost anyone's cupboards. They are common in amazing foods and drinks such as cookies, cake, brownies, ice cream, yoghurt, almost all cereals, sodas, sports drinks, most energy drinks, fruit juice, chocolate milk, most coffee drinks, and even unfortunately protein bars.

"Man, I love protein bars, at least I'm not eating a candy bar, right?" Not exactly, most protein bars have too much sugar in them, which is why they taste so good.

Now you have a basic idea of what sugars are okay in moderation and what sugars you should stay away from as much as possible.

The knowledge of quality foods and drinks in today's society is highly neglected because we have been trained by the big corporations to feed our taste buds instead. We've also been conditioned to emotionally eat, versus consuming what our body really needs in the form of high quality food. Especially in the Unites States. We have become lazy, and frequently turn a blind eye to the harmful foods that we put in our bodies. By harmful I mean putting chemicals and substances in our bodies that we absolutely do not need, and at the same time we neglect the important foods that our body truly needs.

Eating smart and clean is definitely hard work, but once you have a system down it becomes pretty easy. You just have to practice self-discipline like you never have before. Yes, I'll have a bacon cheeseburger with fries, and a coke once in a while but that is not a part of my daily diet. When I want to eat food that doesn't give any nutritional value to my body, I earn it, and keep my body fueled properly the other 98% of the time by eating clean. That way, I feel like I deserve to throw in some junk here and there. Like I said, it is all about discipline and strategy.

Before I end this chapter, there is one more example of sneaky sugars worth mentioning. It is vitamin water. Vitamin water is not water. It is sugar water. If you want vitamins, take a multivitamin with some pure water. By doing that, you will actually absorb more vitamins, and hydrate your body with the water. Yet, people continue to drink vitamin water...and why? Because it tastes good. People use the excuse "but it has vitamins" when the truth is that they drink it because it tastes good, not because it's good for them. It's a sales gimmick. It's a brilliant marketing ploy brought to you by the corporations bottling and selling them. They know how addictive the taste of sugar water can be, and that the masses will keep buying it, drinking it, and telling themselves that it is okay because it has vitamins.

They win, you lose. Don't be a loser.

Don't drink sugar water. Drink plain ole water, it is what your body needs. Which brings us to our next chapter, let's talk about water.

Chapter 2 - Hydrating Your Body

If food is the fuel to your car, water would be the oil. Water makes everything in your body function correctly and run smoothly. Water protects tissues and the spinal cord while it also helps lubricate joints. The human body is made of about 60% water. But a portion of that does get depleted throughout the day from sweating, breathing, peeing, and pooping. I know weird, right? I never thought about it that way either. One thing is for sure; all bodies need water to function properly. Your body will always remind you that it needs water because your brain triggers the body's thirst mechanism, and therefore, you become thirsty. The problem for most people is that they think quenching their thirst can be done with any type of liquid. In theory this does work temporarily because you are no longer feeling thirsty, except you are not really giving your body what it needs. Sure, sugary drinks taste great but drinking them is just succumbing to your taste buds instead of providing the real solution. Your body needs water.

There are endless benefits to drinking water. While I can't tell you all of them, let's pinpoint a few essential ones. Drinking plenty of water will help energize your muscles, and since the goal is to transform your body by building lean mass, this is a very important benefit. Water will also help keep your skin looking good, and it also flushes out your kidneys. Another great tip, if you need assistance controlling calories, water can help with that as well. I've also noticed that drinking a gallon of water a day keeps me from drinking other things that I shouldn't because I'm full of water at all times. These are just a few good examples, and, like I said, there are endless benefits to drinking water.

The idea is to drink at least 128 fluid ounces per day which is 1 gallon.

The hardest part of drinking all that water is to *actually* drink that much liquid. You are most likely not used to drinking a gallon of any liquid in a given day. That seems like a boat load of water to go through in one day doesn't it? Yes, at first if you are not used to it, it may be a little difficult, but there is an easy way to break it down. Start counting your fluid ounces. For example, in a standard small water bottle there are about 17 fluid ounces. You need to drink **eight** of those in a single day. Don't think about the big number, and go slowly through the bottles of water throughout the day until you reach eight.

What I like to do is carry a gallon of water around with me wherever I go throughout the day, which reminds me how much I need to drink. The more I consume, the easier it becomes to carry around. That's just how I do it, but the goal is pretty simple: 128 fluid ounces. It doesn't matter how you break it down, just make sure you drink that amount for best results.

Remember, you only get one body. It's very important to fuel it and lubricate it right. Drink water, and at least a gallon of it every day.

CHAPTER 3 - SUPPLEMENTING YOUR DIET AND TRAINING

Supplements are an essential and fundamental part in the process of transforming the body. Unfortunately, many people waste tremendous amounts of money on them because they don't understand what supplements are and what they really provide. Also, many individuals don't know the difference between which ones are most needed for their body, versus simply buying because the local nutrition store's sales representative said to. People also get sucked into a deceiving advertisement promising magical things that are never going to happen.

You know what I'm talking about. We have all been exposed to shady advertising for ineffectual supplements promising weight loss in a couple weeks by taking their magical pill. Or, "drink this protein powder 3 times a day and you will get all the gains." Yeah, that's not how it works.

A supplement is a substance that helps round out the overall nutritional needs of the body. A supplement enhances an already dialed-in diet, and gives a little extra support that cannot be acquired solely from food. There is no easy way out or cutting corners, no magic pill, shake, drink, or protein bar. And if anyone tells you that they have magical supplements that will give you crazy gains, or make you lose weight, just by taking their product, run from them as fast as you can. Save your money and don't waste your time.

The first step is to follow a strict diet. After that has been mastered, supplements can be added in. Remember, the human body is a machine, and the machine, before anything else, needs fuel and oil to function properly. That being said, when we are looking to push the machine to work harder to either gain lean muscle or to lose body fat, we must give it more fuel and oil for the extra work it is completing. Before anything else, your food and water is always your number one priority.

None of this is to say supplements are bad, a lot of them are actually great for the body and can help it excel. Let's cover how to keep it simple so that you don't waste any more time or money on unnecessary ones. I stick with 6 supplements. Even though there are more that I could additionally take to help, the goal is to keep it as simple, effective, and cost efficient as possible. Supplements are expensive, that is why I feel it is important to only take what you need and save money in the process.

What are the 6 supplements that will aide you to achieve body transformation success? They are as follows:

-Multivitamins

-Omega-3 fatty acids

-Protein powder

- Pre-Workout

-BCAAs (branched-chain amino acids)

-Milk thistle

Now, let's go more into depth. We will start with multivitamins. Multivitamins are a combination of vitamins that are usually found in the foods you eat. However, the reason you want to take multivitamins as an additional supplement is because most people do not consume all of the food that is necessary to meet the recommended amount of vitamins their body needs. There are different ways vitamins can be taken, but the easiest and most common way is to swallow them in pill form daily. There are some liquid vitamins available as well if you don't like swallowing pills. Use whatever form works best for you daily.

The next one is extremely important, and one that many people neglect for some reason. I am talking about omega-3 fatty acids usually in the form of fish oil. Fish oil comes from fatty or oily fish like cod, salmon, krill, sardines, tuna, trout, and herring. Fish oils are a great source of omega-3 fats, vitamin A and vitamin D.

What are the benefits of taking omega-3's? Well, there are a bunch, but here are the important highlights. Fish oils provide omega-3 fats, and that's where the benefits come from. Omega-3 fats give you good heart health, can help reduce 'bad' cholesterol, boosts the good cholesterol, may help reduce weight, supports eye health, helps reduce inflammation, has the potential to make your skin healthier, could help with improved bone health, can help improve symptoms of depression plus anxiety, and honestly, the list goes on and on. This is an essential supplement in my opinion.

Just like multivitamins, fish oil comes in both liquid or pill form. Personally, I suggest the pill form because it is an easy intake of 1-2 pills a day, and you are good to go. Plus, fish oil doesn't necessarily taste fantastic, so drinking it just doesn't sound fun to me. You can choose however you would like to consume it, just make sure that you **do** and that you do it every day. If you can't take fish oils due to allergies, there are alternatives rich in omega-3 like flaxseed oil. Other foods such as chia seeds, spinach, walnuts, and soybeans also contain omega-3 fatty acids.

The next supplement on our list is good ole protein powder. I'm sure you've heard about this one from all of the people you might have talked to about working out or losing weight. Yep, protein powder, this is a great supplement. It's easy to love, especially when it tastes good. Let's dive in.

What's the point of drinking protein shakes, and which one should you buy? Great question because they are not all the same, and there are endless types. There are premade protein shakes that already come bottled, like the ones you find at your local convenience store, and then there are the protein shakes you make at home from actual protein powder. The ones you find pre-made and easily available are usually the ones that taste the best but here's the catch, those are usually pumped full of sugar and fat. Now, our goal is to cut that crap out so we are going to have to get used to the powder instead.

Protein powder itself doesn't always taste as good. That's okay when we remind ourselves that we are fueling our body, not our taste buds. Now, don't get me wrong, there are some powders that taste good, but that is not the industry norm. I personally use the JYM brand, and love the taste (No I don't have a sponsorship with JYM or get paid by them to mention their name, it is just the supplement of my choice for protein powder). My taste buds are different than yours, so you might need to try a few out until you find the one that is best matched for you.

One good thing about buying powder versus pre-made protein shakes is that you save quite a bit of money by buying in bulk and mixing it yourself. The only thing you want to keep in mind when purchasing your protein is to make sure the one you choose is very low in fat and sugar content.

Now, let's discuss crack. This is what makes the fitness world go around. No, I'm not talking about the drug, I'm talking about Pre-Workout. I call it crack because it gives me insane energy, alertness, and crazy pumps at the gym. The insane amount of caffeine concentrated into a tiny little scoop of Pre-Workout sure does make you feel like you're on some sort of drug. Good thing it's legal, and not a street drug because it makes every workout more productive and fun. Okay, enough about how good it is, instead of going on about how much I love it, let me hurry up and tell you more about it. Okay, whew, I'm calm now.

What is Pre-Workout really? And what's in it? And why should you use it? Pre-Workout is just a fancy way of saying "before exercise energy." It usually comes in powder form or a pre-mixed liquid. (Buying the powder will save you money as with protein.) The ingredients that can be found in most Pre-Workout supplements are caffeine, creatine, beta alanine, and L-arginine. There are other chemicals and compounds in Pre-Workout powders that differ from brand to brand, but the main ingredients are the 4 that I listed for you above. There's no need to bore you with hard to read and difficult to understand scientific words and their meanings. I'm going to briefly explain each one of the four main components. Caffeine, as you probably already know, gives you energy. Creatine helps produce energy faster so you can lift harder and more often. It helps you get that extra couple sets or reps in, hence resulting in getting bigger and stronger. Beta alanine increases the amount of work you can do at high intensities. It is also what gives you the "tingle" feeling. If you've taken Pre-Workout, you know what I'm talking about. However, if you've never tried Pre-Workout before, now you will have a heads up. Don't get worried when you try the first full scoop of it. I wish I could be there for that, it's usually pretty funny. Sorry, I get carried away sometimes. L-Argenine allows you to have better blood flow, which is why when you take Pre-Workout, you get a better pump. There are definitely some who say taking Pre-Workout is bad for you, blah-blah-blah. Everything is bad for you. These are the methods that work best for me and many others. It helps my body transformation goals, it gives me better pumps and more energy at the gym. If you rather use a more conservative route, try drinking a couple cups of plain black coffee before your workout, and that might do the trick. I'm pretty passionate about Pre-Workout, but enough on that.

Next up- BCAA'S. BCAA stands for branched chain amino acid. That is an encompassing term for 3 different types of amino acid: leucine, isoleucine, and valine. Now, that sounds like science gibberish and doesn't tell us much. If you want, you can go online and google BCAA's and get a bunch of mumbo jumbo talk, which will most likely look like it's written by and for doctors. At the end of the day, though, most people would rather know what it does without having to decode paragraphs to understand it. Right? I agree, I like keeping things simple, too. For our body transformation goals, what all that stands for, means, or how it breaks down and into what, isn't important. The real question is what does it do? And why should you take it? The answer to these questions is what's going to be important to you in the long run.

Consuming BCAA's during your workout can prevent muscle fatigue from happening quickly, and also help the muscles recover a little faster. BCAA's will also assist in muscle growth over time because of these same reasons. You aren't as tired as fast, and your muscles recover faster so you can push them harder, and more frequently. That's all. I encourage you to wade through all the science talk and research it for yourself.

The final supplement is milk thistle. Milk thistle is a natural herb that has antioxidant and anti-inflammatory properties. It is used to detox the body and usually the liver. Milk thistle can be consumed in a tea form as well as pill, but that takes too much work, in my opinion. Pill form allows us to stick to the easy, fast approach, and can be taken when you take your multivitamins and fish oils. I've read that there are some side effects to consuming too much milk thistle such as diarrhea, nausea, bloating, or upset stomach. Be aware, and speak to your healthcare professional if you have concerns. Personally, I've never had any issues and take two capsules a day. I believe the benefits of cleansing your liver is important for the bodies all around health. Once again, I'm not telling you to take anything; this is the system that I've had the best success with. That covers the basics of the supplements that can help you succeed in your body transformation goals. Remember, the brand of the supplements doesn't necessarily make a difference as long as they are not high in unnecessary sugar or fat. Whatever you do, please don't invest in supplements because you think they will work without doing the work. There is no magic pill that will give anyone the results they want. So please, don't waste your money on quick result promises. Instead, you have to put in the work and use the supplement to enhance your hard work.

CHAPTER 4 - TRAINING YOUR MUSCLES

This step will be fun since I'm guessing you like lifting weights, hence wanting to achieve some extreme body transformation goals such as looking like a shredded bodybuilder. We've already covered how much hard work this process is and how there is no magic pill. By this point, you know that even when you think you've worked hard enough, the work has just begun.

Bodybuilding and dieting is not for everyone. By reading further in this book, and accepting the difficult challenge of working your ass off, that means you are ready to continue.

Now that you know how to fuel and lubricate your machine, it's time to put the beast in action. Weight resistance training is where you put your body to the test. Think of it like a race car; you've been giving it the best oil available and putting in supreme fuel, now you get to see how it performs and what kind of power it puts out.

Since I like to make things simple and efficient, I usually split my body up into 5 different muscles groups to train and focus on each day. These 5 muscle groups will be the following: Your lower body muscles which are your legs and glutes, arms, which include biceps and triceps, chest, shoulders, and back.

By splitting the muscle groups up and training each one on its own day, you are able to give them more attention and focus, getting the most out of each workout. Some people like to mix up different body parts on the same day. I've done this as well, plenty of times; however, I do find that I get the most efficient workouts from separating my muscle groups as listed.

The advanced bodybuilders reading this probably think this is all obvious information, but I like to keep it simple and teach the people who are just getting started.

Now that you have your muscle groups split up, it's important to find the best exercises available for each one. There are many exercises that we could talk about, but then this eBook would never end. Let's shorten it down a little bit. For each muscle group, find 4-5 exercises and do those for about a month. Once you reach the end of that month, look up another 4-5 exercises for each group, and switch it up. When training, try not to do the same exercises for extended amounts of time because your muscles get used to them and will stop developing like you want them to. Different types of exercises can be found either online, from books, or you can always contact me, I would love to help you out.

One question that I frequently hear is "How long should I rest between sets?" This is a great question, and there is not going to be a perfect answer. Personally, my rest intervals between sets will depend on the amount of weight I'm going to be lifting, and the amount of reps I'm going to be doing with that weight. For example, if I'm planning on lifting heavy weight on, let's say, bench press of 8-10 reps, then I will most likely take at least a 3-5 minute break between sets. Five minutes may seem a lot to rest according to some people; however, when I do heavy weights, I prefer to Foam Roll in between sets, which takes time. Some people wait until the end to do that, do what makes the most sense to you. Now, if I'm going to be doing lighter weight, with about 15-20 reps per set, then, as a general rule of thumb, I will rest for about 45 seconds in between sets.

However you do your workouts, whether it is low rep sets with heavy weight or high rep sets with lower weight, always remember to make sure you have your intensity at full throttle. Muscle training, when done right with high intensity, actually burns more fat than cardio exercises. Don't worry, I'm not saying you can skip cardio. Both are needed. Just make sure you do your muscle training workouts with maximum intensity. Speaking of cardio, let's talk about that in the next chapter.

CHAPTER 5 - CARDIO

Cardio stands for cardiovascular exercise. For the sake of keeping things easy and quick, we are going to refer to it as cardio.

What is cardio anyway? Is it just running and getting sweaty? Well, sort of. Cardio is any exercise that raises your heart rate. Why would you want your heart to beat faster? Sounds exhausting, doesn't it? Well it can be, especially if you are doing it right. Most people don't understand that the heart is a muscle. All muscles need to move in order to make them stronger. Since you can't exercise your heart the same way you would your other muscles with weights, you have to get it to beat faster by elevating your heart rate. It is pretty simple, but I've found many people don't think about it this way.

I'll be honest with you, cardio is not my favorite activity. I'd rather lift weights at the gym than get on the treadmill. In order to transform our bodies, we have to do things outside of our comfort zones, and that includes things that aren't as enjoyable, like cardio.

There are many different ways of doing cardio. The most popular one that many people jump to is running. You can run on a track, around your neighborhood, or on a treadmill at the gym. Another good form of cardio is riding a bicycle or use the bike exercise machine at the gym. Swimming is also well liked by many people and is an excellent option. Then there are other cardio exercise machines at the gym like the stair machine or the elliptical machine. I personally only use the stair machine because I feel that it makes your heart work the hardest and gives you the biggest bang for your buck. For example, I can run on a treadmill for an hour with ease and break a little sweat. Now, if I tried to do an hour of stairs, I would be sweating like crazy and would have difficulty completing.

Cardio has many wonderful benefits such as strengthening the heart, reducing mood swings and depression, as well as burning fat. Even though these are all essential for health, we are going to focus on fat burning, which is crucial for body transformation.

The best way to burn fat is to excersise at 60 to 70% of your max heart rate. How do you find out your max heart rate, you ask? Easy, just use this formula (max heart rate = 220 - your age) Let's say you are a thirty-year-old male. Based on the formula, your max heart rate would be 220-30, which is 190. To find 60% of your max rate you multiply 190 by .60 and you get 114. 114 would be 60% of your max heart rate, which is where you would want to be at to burn the most amount of fat while doing your cardio.

How do you know when you are at that number? Most of the cardio equipment at the gyms have heart rate monitors that will show you your rate when you put your hands on a certain part of the equipment, usually a metal piece. Or you can use a Fitbit™, Apple™ watch, or other devices that have the technology to give you heart rate and other body metrics.

With all of the math and different calculations, this stuff can get pretty discouraging. My advice is, don't even worry about the numbers. That little calculation was just a way to give you an idea on how it works, but you don't have to be a mathematician to figure out how to lose fat while doing your cardio. I usually hop on the stairs for 25-30 minutes on level 10 or above. By the time I'm done, I'm sweating like a pig. Also, the stair stepper machine shows you how many calories you are burning, and I try to keep mine at about 250-300.

With your diet dialed in, and your workouts being intense, you won't have to do hours of cardio to get results. A little bit goes a long way. I recommend 25-30 minutes of intense cardio every day, that should be plenty. The key is consistency. Do everything 100%, and work smarter, not harder.

CHAPTER 6 - REST AND RECOVERY

The biggest struggle most people face when trying to live a fit life is consistently making it to the gym. Then there are those, like me and many others, that can't stay away from the gym. We workout six days a week, and when the seventh day comes, we still somehow end up at the gym even though it is a rest day. This is not good. Your body needs rest. No matter how good you feel, how energized you are, or how bad you want to reach your goals – rest is part of the whole picture.

You must rest. Think of a time when you stayed up all night. How did you feel the next day when you had to go to work or the gym? You felt out of it, tired, exhausted, and had trouble staying focused. Your body and mind need sleep for rejuvenation and healing. The same goes for your muscles. They are pushed, pulled, and torn up five to six days a week—on the seventh day those muscles will not give you the same output as they would if they'd had a chance to recover.

What many people don't understand is that your muscles need time to heal, and that this is the period they actually grow. They grow while you are resting them, not when you are working them out. Balance between tearing them up, and then letting them heal is critical. When working hard at the gym, exhausting your muscles, joints, ligaments, and tendons, proper rest time will help them get back to optimal working level.

Eight hours of sleep every night is a good goal to shoot for too when thinking about workout recovery. Now, some people don't have enough time in the day to put aside eight hours. I personally recommend at least eight hours of sleep, but six hours will work if that is all that you can manage. Anything under six hours can put you at risk for potential injury or unnecessary muscle fatigue.

Another key factor in muscle recovery is

stretching. Stretching sucks! Who actually likes stretching? Yes, it's incredibly good for the body and helps it function, as well as move fluidly, but let's be honest, stretching hurts like hell and it can suck. That being said, it doesn't matter how much it hurts, stretching is vital.

As with any routine, consistency is key. Try to incorporate daily stretching into your fitness plan, stretching each one of your bigger muscle groups: back, chest, bicep, tricep, shoulders, legs, and don't forget your glutes. There are a variety of ways to stretch, pick one that works for you and do it daily. I also strongly recommend trying to stretch your muscles out in between sets as well. It will allow you to do more weight with less pain.

Even though there are many different ways of stretching, let's cover one specific one that I don't see many people do at all. They either don't stretch because of time, pain, or simply don't understand the benefits. So, what stretching could I possibly be talking about? It's called foam rolling. What is foam rolling and why should you do it every time you workout?

Foam rolling has become popular in most gyms recently; I'm sure by now you've seen people laying on cylinder shaped objects on the floor making funny faces. You are probably wondering what the hell those people are doing. I know I did for the longest time. After doing some research, and giving it a try, I quickly learned what they hype was all about.

So, what is foam rolling? The official term or name for foam rolling is "self-myofascial release." To make it more understandable and easier to explain to people, I call it "self-massage." It is the best way to release tight muscles. The major muscles you will want to foam roll are usually in your back, legs, and shoulders. It is possible to foam roll your arms too; sometimes I like to do my triceps. But most people stick to rolling the above-mentioned muscle groups.

There are two important things you will want to remember when foam rolling. First, make sure to always go slow. You don't want to roll up and down the foam roller as fast as you can and then call it a day. That's not going to do anything for you. Instead, when beginning, try to find a spot that has built up tension, usually the one that hurts like crazy is the best place to start. When you find that magic spot, try to hold the pressure there, and allow the muscle to slowly release. This is a painful experience, but the more you do it, the more comfortable it will become.

The second thing to pay attention to is the sharpness of pain. If you experience a very sharp sensation, ease away from that area and try to roll a couple of inches away from it. The last thing you want to do is injure yourself. As a trainer, I've seen people ignore the pain and push through it, thinking they are fixing the problem, but in reality, they are making it worse. Foam rolling absolutely should fit into your workout schedule every time. If you are like me, and all you want to do is lift weights as soon as you get to the gym, then definitely pre-plan ahead on how to adjust your routine to incorporate this step. Planning ahead is how we execute an optimal workout experience in our transformation process.

Even after reading and studying about self-myofascial release in my NASM (National Academy of Sport Medicine) certification book, I still had some hesitations. What helped me, and ultimately changed my mind on the whole thing, was something a good trainer friend brought to my attention. He said, "When you foam roll, you spread out your muscle, you can exponentially grow the muscle and get bigger and stronger." That's all I needed to hear. And now I foam roll all the time, I can lift far more weight, with way less pain, than before. Please just trust me and at least try it out. It will work wonders for your recovery.

CHAPTER 7 - PREPARATION FOR SUCCESS

Before I end this book, let's go over one more extremely valuable and useful piece of information. The paramount portion of your body transformation success will depend on how well you prepare for it. Planning, organizing, prepping, cooking, and packaging is where one can truly excel and set themselves up for success. This is also the turning point where one can guarantee less than optimal results.

The choice is yours... I personally always choose success; why else would I even try any diet to begin with? Yes, this may be the boring and toughest portion of it all. However, it must be done with the highest level of persistency to guarantee the success of your diet and eventually the overall achievement of your body transformation. You have to sit down (or you can stand I guess if that is more comfortable) and plan out as well as set up a schedule that you will stick to.

Schedule a day and time to gather, cook, and prepare your food. This might sound like the caveman days, but you have to go gather the critical tools of this preparation, your food. The most difficult part where I see many people struggle is food preparation. Going to the grocery store and preparing your food needs to become a weekly routine. It usually works best if you schedule and commit to a certain time and day of the week for this important step.

Once you have a bunch of food cooked, prepped, and sitting in your refrigerator, the chances that you will actually *eat* that food, instead of something off the diet, will be much higher. In a sense, having those meals prepped and ready can give a sense of obligation; you don't let that effort to go to waste. It is a lot of work to weigh and portion your food correctly based on your diet. For example, some diets will need to be 200 grams of carbs a day, some 150 grams; this is where you will need a trainer to help you set this based on your fitness goals. Unfortunately, I had to find out how to do this by researching the information and then doing the math.

So what is this math I'm now talking about? Let's first discuss why the calculations have to be done, and then I will show you how to apply them in your food prep. If we want to control our carbohydrate intake, we need to know how many carbs we are consuming per meal. Many think this is easy and state the information is on the label. When cooking carbs that don't come with a label such as sweet potatoes, it's difficult to measure your intake. Some carbs, such as rice, do have a label, but even that only tells you how many carbs you get per cup.

Let's say, for your diet, I recommend that you eat six meals at 50 grams of carbs. With that suggestion, we just switched from cups to grams, which can get confusing. One way to make it easier is to calculate it all in grams. This will especially come in handy when it's time to increase or decrease your carb intake.

Unfortunately, the label will not usually tell you weight in grams; this is where you will have to do your own research for each type of food. I've already spent quite a bit of time researching this and want to make it as easy as possible for you. Here is some quick information on a couple of good carb sources to save you some time.

White rice has 28 grams of carbs per 100 grams. To get 50 grams of carbs you would need to eat 180 grams of rice. How did I do the math on that? Simple, I typed in Google™: "how many grams of white rice has 50 grams of carbs in it". That is all. The math isn't complicated; it's just another step to be done. Instead of laying out exact formulas for you here to calculate each one, use a trusted search engine and find the answers quickly. That's part of working smarter, not harder, in this process. Plus, using tried and true resources to get the information faster frees up more time for meal prep.

Another example would be sweet potatoes. There are 20 grams of carbs per 100 grams of baked sweet potatoes. So, to get 50 grams of carbs out of the sweet potatoes you would need to eat 200 grams of it.

The last example I will give you, that many people use as a source of carbs, is quinoa. Quinoa has 26 grams of carbs per 100 grams cooked; its carb count is close to white rice. If you want to get 50 grams of carbs out of quinoa, you would need to eat about 150 grams of it.

If you are the type that would rather do the math and not use a search engine, here is one formula I learned. Once you find out how many carbs come in 100 grams of your selected source, you can plug it into this formula and get the amount you need to consume in grams. Begin by taking the suggested amount of carbs per meal and divide by how many carbs are in 100 grams of your food source. Then multiply that number by 100 to get the weight of your source.

If the goal is to get 50 grams of white rice per meal, and you know that white rice has 28 grams of carbs, then your formula would look like this:

$$50/28=1.78 \text{ then } 1.78 \times 100=178$$

You would need to consume 178 grams of white rice to get 50 grams of carbs. Let's do one more just to make sure you have it down.

It is suggested that you intake 45 grams of carbs per meal. Yams are chosen this time for meal prep. How many grams of yams do you need to eat to make sure you get your 45 grams of carbs?

First, research and find that yams have 29 grams of carbs per 100 grams of yams. Plug it into our formula:

$$45/29=1.55 \text{ then } 1.55 \times 100=155$$

You would need to consume 155 grams of yams to get your 45 grams of carbs per meal.

Did that help? With practice, it becomes a lot easier. I hope this information is useful for you and helps save time. I know I would have saved a ton of time and energy by knowing this stuff from the beginning. I'm happy to share it with others to make their journey easier.

Conclusion

By following these seven simple steps, you can set yourself ahead of 90% of people who are working hard at the gym without seeing results. The main take-away from this book is that all 7 steps must be utilized at the same time. Slacking on any one of them will hinder results. All 7 must be at full throttle with 100% effort for you to see the desired optimal body transformation.

Working out without eating the proper nutrition will not get someone the results they seek. Eating healthy and hoping your muscles develop from your daily activities will not get you there either. Working hard in the gym and trying to replace all your food with supplements will not only take you further away from your goals, but can lead to injury as well. If the goal is to build bulk, doing cardio and simply eating clean won't get you those results. Muscles need to be worked with weight resistance.

All 7 steps tie into each other, and they all must be utilized simultaneously. If you are ready for your body transformation, I would like to challenge you to take these 7 steps, write each one down, then make a list of things that you are going to do to make sure all 7 are completed to the best of your ability.

I know you are ready now. Have fun.

Thanks for reading my book. I can't wait to hear all about your body transformation achievements.

Legal Disclaimer

The information contained in this book is the opinion of the author and is based on the author's personal experiences and observations. The author does not assume any liability whatsoever for the use of or inability to use any or all information contained in this book, and accepts no responsibility for any loss or damages of any kind that may be incurred by the reader as a result of actions arising from the use of information found in this book. Use this information at your own risk.

The author reserves the right to make any changes he deems necessary to future versions of the publication to ensure its accuracy.

www.ingramcontent.com/pod-product-compliance
Lightning Source LLC
Chambersburg PA
CBHW071229280526
45787CB00002B/849